Quit Emotional Eating

An Intervention Without the Fluff

By Dunstamac

The aim of this book is to provide true and credible details on the issue at hand. The publisher is not obliged to offer accounting, lawfully approved, or otherwise qualified services when the book is purchased. A well-versed specialist should be consulted if legal or technological guidance is needed.

The trademarks are used without the permission or backing of the trademark owner, and the trademark is written without the permission or backing of the trademark owner. The trademarks and labels listed in this book are the property of their respective owners, and this text is not associated with them.

Table of contents

<u>Introduction</u>

As a wellness coach, I've done thorough studies on emotional eating and its implications, and I've put together this book with a detailed set of techniques that will hopefully assist you in dealing with your emotional eating habit while also assisting you in being emotionally healthy and independent.

Emotional eating begins at birth as we learn that eating instantly relieves our discomfort (hunger). As humans, we have a propensity to use food to relieve pain. Emotional eating is a pattern in which people use food to help them deal with stressful situations. Several individuals can undergo emotional feeding at any stage in their lives. It - manifests as eating packets of chips when stressed or eating in chocolates after a difficult day at work. However, if emotional eating is done on a daily basis or becomes the primary way a person deals with their emotions, it may have a negative impact on one's health, happiness, and weight. My goal in writing this book is to help you work out how to utilize your inner energies, strengthen your interpersonal relationships, address and resolve stressful stimuli, and show you some emotional eating coping strategies.

To accomplish this goal, I categorized my book into some key parts, each with subsections. In the first segment, I go through some important emotional eating information, followed by subsections on binge eating, emotional and physical hunger, the main causes, and how to cope with them. In the second section, I talk about emotional eating awareness, which includes subsections about why dieting is just a temporary fix for your problems and some solutions that I'll recommend to help you keep hold of your emotional appetite. In the following pages, I'll go through several personal experiences that have helped me regulate emotional eating over time, such as making a journal of your behaviors, maintaining a diet mood diary, and keeping track of your food background. I tie up my book by bringing all of these suggestions together and providing some general guidelines that you might use in a moment of great emotional tension. This coaching book will teach you how to improve your mental health, interact through a multitude of emotional aspects with ease, and cope with feelings effectively without developing emotional eating habits.

<u>Getting on the down-low</u>

By taking a minute to assess your mood, you can begin to reclaim your strength. I've mentioned some key information about emotional eating that you should be aware of. Disturb yourself by finding the answers:

1. What is the concept of binge eating?

BED is characterized by repeated episodes of heavy intake of unusually large amounts of food over a short period of time. These episodes are followed by feelings of guilt, humiliation, and emotional distress. The causes of BED are not well known. Like other eating disorders, it is linked to a variety of environmental, socioeconomic, social, and psychological threats. Overeating compulsively refers to consuming more than is needed. Binge eating disorder is characterized by repeated bouts of compulsive eating that occur even though the person is not hungry. Rapid eating, covert eating, and feeling bad during a binge are also symptoms of bingeing. In the United States, Vyvanse is the only drug licensed to treat binge eating disorder.

1.1. How would it affect you?

BED is related to an increased risk of weight gain and obesity, as well as underlying ailments including diabetes and heart failure. Sleep disturbances, chronic fatigue, mental well-being issues, and a lower standard of living are also potential health risks.

1.2. Difference between Emotional eating and Binge eating

Following are the differences between emotional eating and binge eating.

- Emotional eating is when a person consumes high-carbohydrate, high-calorie foods of little nutritious benefit in reaction to unpleasant emotions such as stress.

- The main distinction between emotional eating and binge eating is the amount of food eaten.

- Emotional eating, like other emotional disorders, is considered to be the product of a combination of causes rather than a particular source.

- Emotional eating, commonly known as panic eating, can show itself in a range of ways.

- Wellness providers check for physical and behavioral health problems when evaluating emotional eating.

- Combating Emotional eating means educating the person on healthy ways to perceive food and build improved eating behaviors (such as conscientious eating), identifying their causes for this behavior, and developing other more appropriate ways to avoid and reduce stress.

- If left unchecked, emotional overeating will contribute to obesity, weight loss issues, and even food abuse.

- Emotional eating can be avoided by reducing depression, eating for nourishment rather than to fix issues, and using constructive approaches to deal with emotions.

1.3. BED is synonymous with bulimia

Fact: Bulimia and BED seem to be identical on the surface. People with the disorders eat excessively and feel anxious, embarrassed, guilty, and out of reach as a consequence of their actions. However, there is one significant distinction between the two scenarios: Bulimia sufferers tend to rid themselves of unnecessary calories by crying, taking laxatives or diuretics (water pills), or over-exercising during a binge.

1.4. What are some of the more popular facts of emotional eating?

There will be certain physical and mental causes for emotional eating. Emotional eating may be triggered by tension or other strong emotions. Coping strategies may assist anyone who is attempting to alleviate more severe symptoms. Just by looking at someone, you can't say whether they have BED. Binge eaters come in a variety of shapes and sizes. What gives that this is possible? Remember that the volume of food and calories are eaten during a "binge" varies from person to person, as does the pace at which calories are burned. Despite this, many individuals with the condition fail to keep a good weight. Obesity is considered to cause around two-thirds of those with the condition.

Other eating disorders, on the other hand, mostly involve women. BED affects both men and women. BED is five times more common in men than any other eating condition. Even if the disorder is related to depressive feelings and increased tension, it's important to note that it's not the same as regular overeating, such as finishing a package of cookies following a split. People with the condition, on the other side, feel tempted to gorge on a daily basis and are unable to regulate their actions.

2. Emotional Hunger vs Physical Hunger

Can you get hungry right away while you're down? Emotional appetite is popular, but it is not the same as physical hunger.

2.1. What is Physical Hunger?

Physical hunger is when the body exhibits hunger signs. And you stop eating when you're uncomfortably whole. Stomach grumbling, feeling weekly or fatigued, hypoglycemia, and feeling lightheaded are all common physical hunger symptoms.

2.2. Stress's physical effect: Increased Food Cravings

Stress is a mental disorder that affects a person's eating and sleeping habits, as well as how they feel about themselves and how they think about problems. Significant depression, dysthymia, and bipolar disorder are the three main forms of depression (also called manic-depressive disease).

There are many physical reasons why a person can overeat as a result of stress and intense emotions:

- **High cortisol levels:** Tension induces the appetite to reduce in order for the body to cope with the crisis. If the stress does not subside, the hormone cortisol is released. Cortisol increases appetite, which may contribute to overeating.

- **Cravings:** Stress-induced rises in cortisol levels can exacerbate food cravings for sweets or unhealthy food.

Increased appetite hormones are often linked to fatigue which may contribute to fast food abuse.

- **Gender:** Several studies show that females are more likely than males to use food to deal with stress, while men are far more likely to smoke or drink alcohol.

2.3. What is emotional eating?

Instead of satisfying the needs of the body, emotional hunger is all about eliminating depressive emotions by eating sugary snacks or other calming foods. Comfort foods are usually heavy in sugar and carbohydrates. Anything from work stress to financial issues may be at the center of emotional eating.

2.4. Does emotional eating occur suddenly or gradually?

Emotional deprivation seems to occur suddenly and without warning, and it appears to be immediate. Physical starvation is therefore not as sudden or surprising as it is when a person hasn't eaten for a long time.

2.5. Do you have an addiction to a particular food?

Physical hunger is usually associated with junk food cravings or something unhealthy. Someone who is genuinely starving will still eat something, but anyone who is mentally stressed would want something unusual, such as fries or pizza.

2.6. Is there such a thing as mindless food consumption?

When people consume without paying attention to what they're drinking or eating, it's known as mindless eating.

One example is eating a whole bowl of ice cream while watching TV, despite not planning to eat too much. When it comes to emotional feeding, this is a normal phenomenon, as opposed to consuming out of hunger.

2.7. Is hunger perceived in the head or in the stomach?

The stomach may not be the cause of emotional hunger, such as a rumbling and growling stomach. Emotional hunger tends to begin when a person demonstrates an urge or a need for something important to eat.

2.8. Are there any feelings of regret or shame during emotional feeding?

By giving in to temptation or eating due to stress, it may trigger feelings of regret, remorse, or guilt. These responses tend to be linked to emotional hunger. Physical hunger, on the other hand, supplies the body with the nutrients or calories it needs to function and is not associated with negative feelings.

3. Emotional Triggers

On any given day, you are likely to encounter a spectrum of emotions, including excitement, unease, frustration, enjoyment, and dissatisfaction. These rules often extend to real-life situations, such as meeting with your boss, talking with a pal about current affairs, or seeing your partner.

The following are examples of situations that can elicit strong emotions

- Betrayed trust
- Inequitable treatment
- Standards that were not fulfilled
- A sense of helplessness or a shortage of supervision
- Left out or forgotten
- Critique or allegation
- Uncomfortable or unneeded thoughts
- The feeling of being surrounded or excessively wanted
- Confusion
- Loss of liberty
- Being turned down

The way you respond to such events can change your emotional status and the circumstances of the situation.

3.1. How to Recognize Yours

Emotional triggers are present in almost all, but they vary in appearance from individual to person. They can include memories of negative past encounters, unpleasant topics, other people's remarks or behavior, or your own behaviors.

<u>Awareness</u>

And how would we change anything if we aren't aware of it? As a fitness instructor, I'll share few tips about how to become more mindful of your food patterns and how they affect your mood.

Here are few suggestions for you to remember.

1. The Food History

When you're depressed, do you find yourself reaching for snacks? It's normal for people to look to food for warmth. That is a characteristic of emotional eating. On the other side, physical hunger occurs as the body sends you signals that you are actually starving. Worse, we don't often switch to food to satisfy our thirst. We gorge on such items even too often to alleviate discomfort or other messes. Find out which food cravings will throw your diet off. Food cravings are harmful to the waistline, whether they are creamy or crunchy, sweet or salty. For your health's sake, learn to make healthier dietary decisions.

Keep a journal of all that comes to mind, as well as a record of your emotional past.

Question	Your Response
What was it like at your house during mealtime?	
Before going to classes, what did you have for breakfast?	

Is it true that the whole family ate dinner together?

____

What was it like for you?

____

Were you ever complimented for your eating skills?

____

Have you ever been chastised for being a picky eater?

____

Were you hungry all of the time or just occasionally?

____

What are large family get-together's, such as holidays?

____

What are the plans for the holidays?

____

Did you seek solace from food?

____

When did it all begin?

____

When you were overweight?

____

When did they first start?

____

If you have some particular things that you crave?

____

When did this begin?

____

What did your caregivers think about your dietary habits?

____

What were the messages you sent yourself about your eating habits?

____

Have you developed a binge eating problem?

____

If so, when do you think that would happen?

____

Do you ever feel out of balance when it comes to food?

____

If that's the case, where did it start?

Has diet been a healthy haven for you?

When did it begin?

Do you have any children?

What was your reaction to them in terms of food?

How did the kids handle mealtime?

Are you now doing the "See Food" diet: see it, eat it!

Are you bombarded with health and food commercials?

If that's the case, which one is it?

____

Will you refrain from consuming such foods (junk food)?

____

As long as it is not in focus?

____

If you have a habit of paying for your meals?

____

Did you go on a diet? Effectively or unsuccessfully?

____

2. The Food-Mood Diary

One of the first steps to increase consciousness is to pay close attention to what you consume. If you're reading this after you've already consumed a meal or two, you should begin right now. What did you have for dinner? Assess the day to the highest possible norm. When are you going to do it? Are you aware of any stimulating occurrences or emotions when you eat? If you continue to do this, you may become more conscious of the triggering experiences and emotions that will cause you to feed.

("Fill in the sheet any time you consume anything in the next thirty days (yes, even one nibble of something counts)").

Time/Date	Food	Event	Mood

3. Your Journal

Keeping a journal will help you deal with mental eating disorders in a therapeutic manner. I maintained a journal of my private thoughts and emotions for several years. I always began a page by writing, "I don't know what to write about today." My pen was gliding over the paper in a few minutes, leaving a trail of words in its path. I let the words flow freely on the paper, feeling everything that was bubbling up inside of me. I didn't worry about spelling or punctuation; I just let my hand keep writing until it was exhausted. The time was spent, but it was spent more happily. Writing has been extremely therapeutic for me. For a couple of months, keep a diet journal. Create a note of what you consume and why you eat everything. It will assist you in defining your patterns. You may find, for example, that you crave a sweet snack to help you through the mid-afternoon energy low. It's important to keep track of how you felt when you wanted to eat, particularly if you ate when you weren't hungry. Were you exhausted? Are you feeling tense?

Instead of eating your emotions, start writing them down in a journal. You can write whatever you want and keep writing until you have a clear picture of yourself. When you write for at least 15 minutes every day, you'll soon discover the magic of keeping a journal!

Your journal

4. Diets are a self-contained, temporary cure

The irony is that these interventions are ineffective because the deeper issues are not addressed. Diets, for example, fail because they focus solely on the level of shallow behavior. People are led to believe that if they just lose weight, their lives will improve, their depression will subside, and that once the diet is over, they will magically become relaxed around food. If you're reading this, you've probably already admitted to yourself that dieting only makes things worse. Abstinence from food addiction entails ceasing to engage in the behaviors associated with your eating disorder, such as binge eating, obsessing over food, limiting, and all other behaviors associated with your specific type of food or eating addict.

5. The Union

Whatever you do, whether it's your dietary patterns, how you drink everything you buy, or how you feel for your body, happens for whatever purpose. It's called the superficial stage because it's not the cause of the problem; although it is a problem, it's just what's closer to the top. The issue isn't one of food. The issues arise from the way food is consumed. If you never reform your habits, you'll just be able to change them for a short time. To have a better understanding of what motivates you to use food the way you do, dig a little deeper.

<u>Self-Care</u>

1. Breathing slowly

If you're deliriously cheerful or so sad that you can't talk, the force of a deep breath has a lot to say. Slowing things down and paying attention to what's going on won't help the feelings go away fast (and realize, that is not the goal).

- **Take a deep breath in slowly:** The diaphragm, not the lung, takes deep breaths. Visualize your breath slowly rising from deep inside your belly button. Yeah, you've got it. Hold the breath for three counts, and slowly release it.

- **Think of the mantra**: Hearing a mantra, such as "I am calm" or "I am peaceful," maybe calming to certain people.

2. Offer Some Space to Yourself

Taking the time away from intense feelings, in my opinion, can help you ensure that you are listening to them rationally. This chasm could be emotional, such as quitting an upsetting circumstance. However, by occupying yourself, you will also develop self-esteem.

While you don't want to totally suppress or stop feelings, it's not harmful to distract yourself while you're in a better mood to deal with them. Just make sure you're on your way back to them. Healthy distractions are just temporary.

3. Try Some Distractions

Take a hike, enjoy a good show, talk to a loved one, pet the cat for a few minutes, catch as much sleep as possible, create time for friends to chat (and laugh), exercise, spend time with loved ones, and find time for relaxation and hobbies.

If you've figured out what you're doing, you'll be able to approach and learn from those emotions that are more well established.

4. Meditation

If you aren't currently seeing a psychiatrist, that might be one of the better choices for coping with extreme feelings. Meditation will help you develop a deeper view of your emotions and experiences. When meditating, you teach yourself to calm down with those feelings, to notice them without judging yourself or trying to alter or remove them.

It can foster emotional regulation by teaching you to understand all of your feelings, as mentioned above. Meditation helps you to develop your acceptance skills. It also has other benefits, such as assisting you in relaxing and sleeping well.

5. Self-Care Activity

It is important that we have a greater understanding of ourselves! What self-care habits would you love to incorporate into your everyday routine? Any suggestions: Relax in a hot bath with candles or bath salts. Only enjoy a nice time. Pour yourself a cup of coffee and sit back for five minutes. For ten minutes, don't do something until you've had a cup of tea. Make a list right now.

6. Identify Toxic Relationship

When it comes to managing emotional stimuli, you have a lot of leverage. Your answers are not the liability of someone else. They are, moreover, responsible for their behavior, which can lead you to feel upset. So, as a coach, my advice is to recognize those individuals and stay away from them.

7. Supporting Group

"Finding supporting people or forming a social network satisfies our fundamental desire to belong."

Start recognizing the people who can help you. These are the ones who can listen to you without passing judgment and will be there to support you.

First, you have to list down the qualities you are seeking in your support group as following:

1. ------------------------------	6. -------------------------------
2. ------------------------------	7. -----------------------------
3. ------------------------------	8. ------------------------------

4. ----------------------------------   9. ----------------------------------

5. ----------------------------------   10. ----------------------------------

Then list the people who fit these qualities, and list them as follows:

1. --

2. --

3. --

4. --

5. --

<u>Conclusion</u>

Putting all of the above into consideration, the most common causes cited by people are loneliness, schedules, exhaustion, and social pressures. The first phase in overcoming emotional eating is to understand the causes and circumstances that arise in one's life. Holding a food diary or document may help pinpoint periods that someone is overeating due to emotional hunger rather than physical hunger. Anyone may gain insight into their eating patterns by tracking their behavior.

They'd like to brainstorm suggestions about how to fix their proven causes next. Anyone who eats when stressed, for example, might start learning a new book that sounds fascinating or starting a new challenging task. To help themselves deal with their feelings, anyone who consumes due to stress can prefer to meditate, rest, or go for a walk. Anyone who emotionally eats can attempt to call a friend, take their dog for a walk, or schedule an adventure to deal with their "bad feelings" while they are depressed. Try using all of the above techniques to see how the emotional eating preferences shift.